"*I choose to happiness over mi...*"

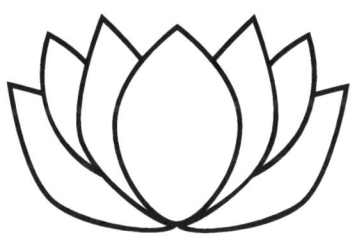

This Journal Belongs To

_____

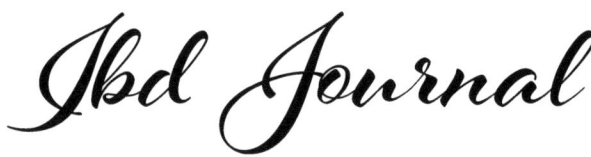

PAIN & SYMPTOMS TRACKER WITH FOOD LOG

When you have a digestive disorder like **IBD (Ulcerative Colitis or Crohn's Disease), Celiac Disease, IBS (Irritable Bowel Syndrome),** or any other digestive disease, you understand the importance of keeping a daily food diary to track food intakes, symptoms, and pain levels to identify your digestive triggers and keep flares to a minimum.

Keeping a journal and tracking your symptoms and pain levels can be extremely beneficial. Whether you're trying to get an accurate diagnosis, adjust your treatment plan, or identify trends in your overall health and wellness, keeping a symptoms diary can be a useful tool for communicating with your health care providers.

Each day, use the tracking pages to log down the severity of your pain and its symptoms, medication, sleep, and mood. A daily food log is also provided to keep track of your food intake and symptoms associated with it.

It also includes pages to record your doctor's appointment and reason for visit, making it easier to follow up for your medical check-ups.

This symptom tracking journal is ideal for assisting you in getting a handle on things, bringing your illness to a successful conclusion, and living the healthiest life possible.

© 2021 BLACK FOREST PUBLICATIONS
ALL RIGHTS ARE RESERVED.

INSURANCE DETAILS

Company: _____

Plan Type: _____

ID Number: _____

Contact Person: _____

Phone Number: _____

Email Number: _____

MEDICAL CONTACTS

Name: _____

Contact Person: _____

Phone Number: _____

Email Number: _____

Notes: _____

Date:_____

S M T W T F S

Meals

Exercise:_____

Total Calories Burned:_____

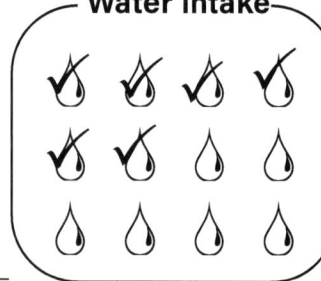
Water Intake

	Time	Food & Drinks	Symptoms	Triggers	Notes
Breakfast	7:30 Am	Egg Sandwich Orange juice	All good.		

Carb:_____ Fat:_____ Total Sugar:_____
Fiber:_____ Protein:_____ Calories: 300 cal

Snack					

Carb:_____ Fat:_____ Total Sugar:_____
Fiber:_____ Protein:_____ Calories:_____

Lunch					

Example

Carb:_____ Fat:_____ Total Sugar:_____
Fiber:_____ Protein:_____ Calories:_____

Snack					

Carb:_____ Fat:_____ Total Sugar:_____
Fiber:_____ Protein:_____ Calories:_____

Dinner					

Carb:_____ Fat:_____ Total Sugar:_____
Fiber:_____ Protein:_____ Calories:_____

Pain

Where does it hurt?

How severe is the pain?

1   (2)   3   4   5

Headache but manageable
_____

Did you take any medication? _Paracetamol_

Did it help? _Yes_

Time	Symptoms	Triggers

Example

Other Symptoms Tracker

- ○ Pain
- ✓ Constipation
- ○ Bleeding
- ○ Fatigue
- ○ Bloating
- ○ Sweats
- ○ Cramping
- ○ Others:_____
- ○ _____

Bowel Movement

BM#1	BM#2	BM#3	BM#4
BM#5	BM#6	BM#7	BM#8

Energy Level ○ Low ✓ Med ○ High
Activity Level ○ Low ○ Med ✓ High
Mood   ○ Sad ✓ Good ○ Happy

Sleep ○ 😐 ✓ 🙂

Notes:
_____

Doctor's Appointment

DOCTOR: _Dr .. ABC_____
CLINIC: _XYZ Clinic_____
DATE: _20th of March, 20XX_____
REASON: _Lower Back Pain._____
RESULT: _XXXX.......Etc._____

_____

DOCTOR:_____
CLINIC:_____
DATE:_____
REASON:_____
RESULT:_____

Example

_____

DOCTOR:_____
CLINIC:_____
DATE:_____
REASON:_____
RESULT:_____

_____

DOCTOR:_____
CLINIC:_____
DATE:_____
REASON:_____
RESULT:_____

_____

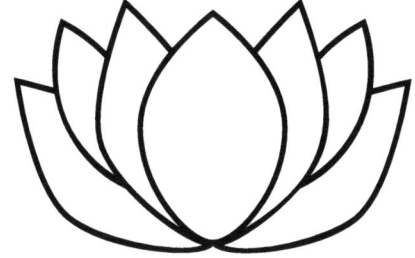

Table Of Contents

Appointment Log 08

Daily Food Log & Symptoms Tracker 12

Doctor's Appointment

DOCTOR: _____
CLINIC: _____
DATE: _____
REASON: _____
RESULT: _____
_____

DOCTOR: _____
CLINIC: _____
DATE: _____
REASON: _____
RESULT: _____
_____

DOCTOR: _____
CLINIC: _____
DATE: _____
REASON: _____
RESULT: _____
_____

DOCTOR: _____
CLINIC: _____
DATE: _____
REASON: _____
RESULT: _____
_____

Doctor's Appointment

DOCTOR: _____
CLINIC: _____
DATE: _____
REASON: _____
RESULT: _____
_____

DOCTOR: _____
CLINIC: _____
DATE: _____
REASON: _____
RESULT: _____
_____

DOCTOR: _____
CLINIC: _____
DATE: _____
REASON: _____
RESULT: _____
_____

DOCTOR: _____
CLINIC: _____
DATE: _____
REASON: _____
RESULT: _____
_____

Doctor's Appointment

DOCTOR: _____
CLINIC: _____
DATE: _____
REASON: _____
RESULT: _____
_____

DOCTOR: _____
CLINIC: _____
DATE: _____
REASON: _____
RESULT: _____
_____

DOCTOR: _____
CLINIC: _____
DATE: _____
REASON: _____
RESULT: _____
_____

DOCTOR: _____
CLINIC: _____
DATE: _____
REASON: _____
RESULT: _____
_____

Doctor's Appointment

DOCTOR: _____
CLINIC: _____
DATE: _____
REASON: _____
RESULT: _____

_____

DOCTOR: _____
CLINIC: _____
DATE: _____
REASON: _____
RESULT: _____

_____

DOCTOR: _____
CLINIC: _____
DATE: _____
REASON: _____
RESULT: _____

_____

DOCTOR: _____
CLINIC: _____
DATE: _____
REASON: _____
RESULT: _____

_____

Date:_____

S M T W T F S

Meals

Exercise:_____

Total Calories Burned:_____

Water Intake

	Time	Food & Drinks	Symptoms	Triggers	Notes
Breakfast					

Carb:_____, Fat:_____, Total Sugar:_____,
Fiber: _____, Protein:_____, Calories:_____

Snack					

Carb:_____, Fat:_____, Total Sugar:_____,
Fiber: _____, Protein:_____, Calories:_____

Lunch					

Carb:_____, Fat:_____, Total Sugar:_____,
Fiber: _____, Protein:_____, Calories:_____

Snack					

Carb:_____, Fat:_____, Total Sugar:_____,
Fiber: _____, Protein:_____, Calories:_____

Dinner					

Carb:_____, Fat:_____, Total Sugar:_____,
Fiber: _____, Protein:_____, Calories:_____

Pain

Where does it hurt?

How severe is the pain?

1   2   3   4   5

_____
_____

Did you take any medication? _____

Did it help? _____

Time	Symptoms	Triggers

Other Symptoms Tracker

- ○ Pain
- ○ Constipation
- ○ Bleeding
- ○ Fatigue
- ○ Bloating
- ○ Sweats
- ○ Cramping
- ○ Others:_____
- ○ _____

Bowel Movement

BM#1	BM#2	BM#3	BM#4
BM#5	BM#6	BM#7	BM#8

Energy Level ○ Low ○ Med ○ High
Activity Level ○ Low ○ Med ○ High
Mood ○ Sad ○ Good ○ Happy

Sleep ○ 😐 ○ 🙂

Notes: _____

Date:_____

S M T W T F S

Meals

Exercise:_____

Total Calories Burned:_____

Water Intake

	Time	Food & Drinks	Symptoms	Triggers	Notes
Breakfast					

Carb:_____, Fat:_____, Total Sugar:_____,
Fiber: _____, Protein:_____, Calories:_____

Snack					

Carb:_____, Fat:_____, Total Sugar:_____,
Fiber: _____, Protein:_____, Calories:_____

Lunch					

Carb:_____, Fat:_____, Total Sugar:_____,
Fiber: _____, Protein:_____, Calories:_____

Snack					

Carb:_____, Fat:_____, Total Sugar:_____,
Fiber: _____, Protein:_____, Calories:_____

Dinner					

Carb:_____, Fat:_____, Total Sugar:_____,
Fiber: _____, Protein:_____, Calories:_____

Pain

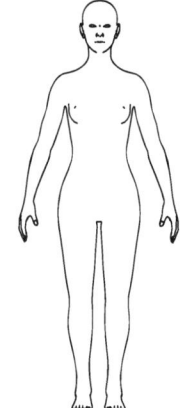

Where does it hurt?

 How severe is the pain?

    1   2   3   4   5

_____

_____

Did you take any medication?_____

Did it help?_____

Time	Symptoms	Triggers

Other Symptoms Tracker

- ○ Pain
- ○ Constipation
- ○ Bleeding
- ○ Fatigue
- ○ Bloating
- ○ Sweats
- ○ Cramping
- ○ Others:_____
- ○ _____

Bowel Movement

BM#1	BM#2	BM#3	BM#4
BM#5	BM#6	BM#7	BM#8

Energy Level ○ Low ○ Med ○ High   **Sleep**

Activity Level ○ Low ○ Med ○ High

Mood ○ Sad ○ Good ○ Happy ○   ○

Notes:_____

Date:_____

S M T W T F S

Meals

Exercise:_____

Total Calories Burned:_____

Water Intake

	Time	Food & Drinks	Symptoms	Triggers	Notes
Breakfast					

Carb:_____, Fat:_____, Total Sugar:_____,
Fiber: _____, Protein:_____, Calories:_____

| **Snack** | | | | | |

Carb:_____, Fat:_____, Total Sugar:_____,
Fiber: _____, Protein:_____, Calories:_____

| **Lunch** | | | | | |

Carb:_____, Fat:_____, Total Sugar:_____,
Fiber: _____, Protein:_____, Calories:_____

| **Snack** | | | | | |

Carb:_____, Fat:_____, Total Sugar:_____,
Fiber: _____, Protein:_____, Calories:_____

| **Dinner** | | | | | |

Carb:_____, Fat:_____, Total Sugar:_____,
Fiber: _____, Protein:_____, Calories:_____

Pain

Where does it hurt?

How severe is the pain?

1   2   3   4   5

_____
_____

Did you take any medication? _____

Did it help? _____

Time	Symptoms	Triggers

Other Symptoms Tracker

- O Pain
- O Constipation
- O Bleeding
- O Fatigue
- O Bloating
- O Sweats
- O Cramping
- O Others: _____
- O _____

Bowel Movement

BM#1	BM#2	BM#3	BM#4
BM#5	BM#6	BM#7	BM#8

Energy Level O Low O Med O High
Activity Level O Low O Med O High
Mood O Sad O Good O Happy

Sleep O O

Notes: _____

Date:____

S M T W T F S

Meals

Exercise:_____

Total Calories Burned:_____

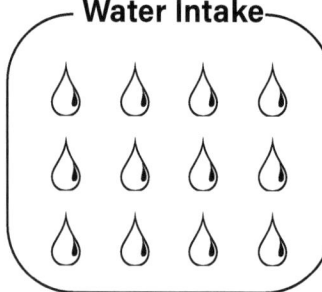
Water Intake

	Time	Food & Drinks	Symptoms	Triggers	Notes
Breakfast					

Carb:_____, Fat:_____, Total Sugar:_____,
Fiber: _____, Protein:_____, Calories:_____

Snack					

Carb:_____, Fat:_____, Total Sugar:_____,
Fiber: _____, Protein:_____, Calories:_____

Lunch					

Carb:_____, Fat:_____, Total Sugar:_____,
Fiber: _____, Protein:_____, Calories:_____

Snack					

Carb:_____, Fat:_____, Total Sugar:_____,
Fiber: _____, Protein:_____, Calories:_____

Dinner					

Carb:_____, Fat:_____, Total Sugar:_____,
Fiber: _____, Protein:_____, Calories:_____

Pain

Where does it hurt?

 How severe is the pain?

    1   2   3   4   5

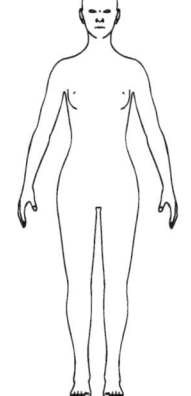

_____
_____

Did you take any medication?_____

Did it help?_____

Time	Symptoms	Triggers

Other Symptoms Tracker

- ○ Pain
- ○ Constipation
- ○ Bleeding
- ○ Fatigue
- ○ Bloating
- ○ Sweats
- ○ Cramping
- ○ Others:_____
- ○ _____

Bowel Movement

BM#1	BM#2	BM#3	BM#4
BM#5	BM#6	BM#7	BM#8

				Sleep
Energy Level	○ Low	○ Med	○ High	
Activity Level	○ Low	○ Med	○ High	○ 😐 ○ 🙂
Mood	○ Sad	○ Good	○ Happy	

Notes: _____

19

Date:_____

S M T W T F S

Meals

Exercise:_____

Total Calories Burned:_____

Water Intake

	Time	Food & Drinks	Symptoms	Triggers	Notes
Breakfast					

Carb:_____, Fat:_____, Total Sugar:_____,
Fiber: _____, Protein:_____, Calories:_____

Snack					

Carb:_____, Fat:_____, Total Sugar:_____,
Fiber: _____, Protein:_____, Calories:_____

Lunch					

Carb:_____, Fat:_____, Total Sugar:_____,
Fiber: _____, Protein:_____, Calories:_____

Snack					

Carb:_____, Fat:_____, Total Sugar:_____,
Fiber: _____, Protein:_____, Calories:_____

Dinner					

Carb:_____, Fat:_____, Total Sugar:_____,
Fiber: _____, Protein:_____, Calories:_____

Pain

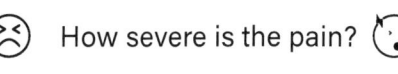 How severe is the pain?

1   2   3   4   5

Where does it hurt?

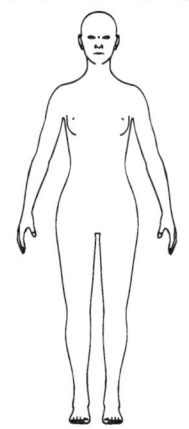

_____
_____

Did you take any medication?_____

Did it help?_____

Time	Symptoms	Triggers

Other Symptoms Tracker

- O Pain
- O Constipation
- O Bleeding
- O Fatigue
- O Bloating
- O Sweats
- O Cramping
- O Others:_____
- O _____

Bowel Movement

BM#1	BM#2	BM#3	BM#4
BM#5	BM#6	BM#7	BM#8

Energy Level O Low   O Med   O High

Activity Level O Low   O Med   O High

Mood O Sad   O Good   O Happy

Sleep O   O

Notes: _____

21

Date:_____

S M T W T F S

Meals

Exercise:_____

Total Calories Burned:_____

Water Intake

	Time	Food & Drinks	Symptoms	Triggers	Notes
Breakfast					

Carb:_____, Fat:_____, Total Sugar:_____,
Fiber: _____, Protein:_____, Calories:_____

Snack					

Carb:_____, Fat:_____, Total Sugar:_____,
Fiber: _____, Protein:_____, Calories:_____

Lunch					

Carb:_____, Fat:_____, Total Sugar:_____,
Fiber: _____, Protein:_____, Calories:_____

Snack					

Carb:_____, Fat:_____, Total Sugar:_____,
Fiber: _____, Protein:_____, Calories:_____

Dinner					

Carb:_____, Fat:_____, Total Sugar:_____,
Fiber: _____, Protein:_____, Calories:_____

Pain

Where does it hurt?

 How severe is the pain?

1   2   3   4   5

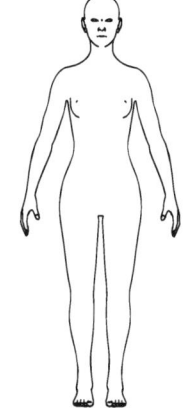

_____

_____

Did you take any medication?_____

Did it help?_____

Time	Symptoms	Triggers

Other Symptoms Tracker

- ○ Pain
- ○ Constipation
- ○ Bleeding
- ○ Fatigue
- ○ Bloating
- ○ Sweats
- ○ Cramping
- ○ Others:_____
- ○ _____

Bowel Movement

BM#1	BM#2	BM#3	BM#4
BM#5	BM#6	BM#7	BM#8

Energy Level   ○ Low   ○ Med   ○ High

Activity Level   ○ Low   ○ Med   ○ High

Mood   ○ Sad   ○ Good   ○ Happy

Sleep   ○   ○ 🙂

Notes:
_____

Date: _____

S M T W T F S

Meals

Exercise: _____

Total Calories Burned: _____

Water Intake

	Time	Food & Drinks	Symptoms	Triggers	Notes
Breakfast					

Carb:_____, Fat:_____, Total Sugar:_____,
Fiber: _____, Protein:_____, Calories:_____

Snack					

Carb:_____, Fat:_____, Total Sugar:_____,
Fiber: _____, Protein:_____, Calories:_____

Lunch					

Carb:_____, Fat:_____, Total Sugar:_____,
Fiber: _____, Protein:_____, Calories:_____

Snack					

Carb:_____, Fat:_____, Total Sugar:_____,
Fiber: _____, Protein:_____, Calories:_____

Dinner					

Carb:_____, Fat:_____, Total Sugar:_____,
Fiber: _____, Protein:_____, Calories:_____

Pain

Where does it hurt?

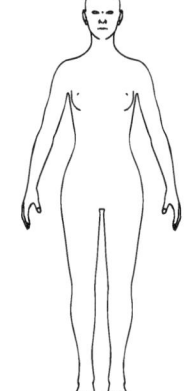

 How severe is the pain?

1   2   3   4   5

_____
_____

Did you take any medication?_____

Did it help?_____

Time	Symptoms	Triggers

Other Symptoms Tracker

- O Pain
- O Constipation
- O Bleeding
- O Fatigue
- O Bloating
- O Sweats
- O Cramping
- O Others:_____
- O _____

Bowel Movement

BM#1	BM#2	BM#3	BM#4
BM#5	BM#6	BM#7	BM#8

Energy Level   O Low   O Med   O High   **Sleep**
Activity Level O Low   O Med   O High
Mood   O Sad   O Good O Happy   O 😐   O 🙂

Notes: _____

25

Date:____

S M T W T F S

Meals

Exercise:_____

Total Calories Burned:_____

Water Intake

	Time	Food & Drinks	Symptoms	Triggers	Notes
Breakfast					

Carb:_____, Fat:_____, Total Sugar:_____,
Fiber: _____, Protein:_____, Calories:_____

Snack					

Carb:_____, Fat:_____, Total Sugar:_____,
Fiber: _____, Protein:_____, Calories:_____

Lunch					

Carb:_____, Fat:_____, Total Sugar:_____,
Fiber: _____, Protein:_____, Calories:_____

Snack					

Carb:_____, Fat:_____, Total Sugar:_____,
Fiber: _____, Protein:_____, Calories:_____

Dinner					

Carb:_____, Fat:_____, Total Sugar:_____,
Fiber: _____, Protein:_____, Calories:_____

Pain

 How severe is the pain?

1   2   3   4   5

_____
_____

Did you take any medication?_____

Did it help?_____

Where does it hurt?

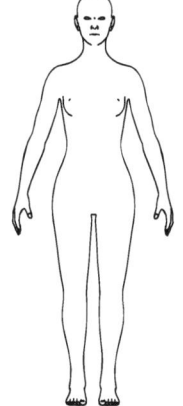

Time	Symptoms	Triggers

Other Symptoms Tracker

- ○ Pain
- ○ Constipation
- ○ Bleeding
- ○ Fatigue
- ○ Bloating
- ○ Sweats
- ○ Cramping
- ○ Others:_____
- ○ _____

Bowel Movement

BM#1	BM#2	BM#3	BM#4
BM#5	BM#6	BM#7	BM#8

Energy Level   ○ Low   ○ Med   ○ High
Activity Level   ○ Low   ○ Med   ○ High
Mood   ○ Sad   ○ Good   ○ Happy

Sleep   ○ 😐   ○ 🙂

Notes: _____

Date: _____

S M T W T F S

Meals

Exercise: _____

Total Calories Burned: _____

Water Intake

	Time	Food & Drinks	Symptoms	Triggers	Notes
Breakfast					

Carb:_____, Fat:_____, Total Sugar:_____,
Fiber: _____, Protein:_____, Calories:_____

Snack					

Carb:_____, Fat:_____, Total Sugar:_____,
Fiber: _____, Protein:_____, Calories:_____

Lunch					

Carb:_____, Fat:_____, Total Sugar:_____,
Fiber: _____, Protein:_____, Calories:_____

Snack					

Carb:_____, Fat:_____, Total Sugar:_____,
Fiber: _____, Protein:_____, Calories:_____

Dinner					

Carb:_____, Fat:_____, Total Sugar:_____,
Fiber: _____, Protein:_____, Calories:_____

Pain

☹ How severe is the pain? 😮

1   2   3   4   5

_____
_____

Did you take any medication? _____

Did it help? _____

Where does it hurt?

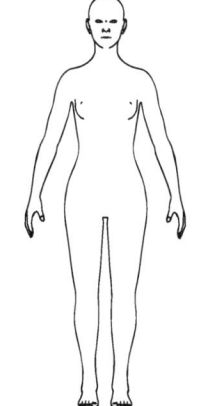

Time	Symptoms	Triggers

Other Symptoms Tracker

- ○ Pain
- ○ Constipation
- ○ Bleeding
- ○ Fatigue
- ○ Bloating
- ○ Sweats
- ○ Cramping
- ○ Others:_____
- ○ _____

Bowel Movement

BM#1	BM#2	BM#3	BM#4
BM#5	BM#6	BM#7	BM#8

Energy Level ○ Low ○ Med ○ High

Activity Level ○ Low ○ Med ○ High

Mood ○ Sad ○ Good ○ Happy

Sleep ○   ○

Notes: _____

Date:_____

S M T W T F S

Meals

Exercise:_____

Total Calories Burned:_____

Water Intake

	Time	Food & Drinks	Symptoms	Triggers	Notes
Breakfast					

Carb:_____, Fat:_____, Total Sugar:_____,
Fiber: _____, Protein:_____, Calories:_____

	Time	Food & Drinks	Symptoms	Triggers	Notes
Snack					

Carb:_____, Fat:_____, Total Sugar:_____,
Fiber: _____, Protein:_____, Calories:_____

	Time	Food & Drinks	Symptoms	Triggers	Notes
Lunch					

Carb:_____, Fat:_____, Total Sugar:_____,
Fiber: _____, Protein:_____, Calories:_____

	Time	Food & Drinks	Symptoms	Triggers	Notes
Snack					

Carb:_____, Fat:_____, Total Sugar:_____,
Fiber: _____, Protein:_____, Calories:_____

	Time	Food & Drinks	Symptoms	Triggers	Notes
Dinner					

Carb:_____, Fat:_____, Total Sugar:_____,
Fiber: _____, Protein:_____, Calories:_____

Pain

Where does it hurt?

How severe is the pain?

1   2   3   4   5

_____
_____

Did you take any medication? _____

Did it help? _____

Time	Symptoms	Triggers

Other Symptoms Tracker

- ○ Pain
- ○ Constipation
- ○ Bleeding
- ○ Fatigue
- ○ Bloating
- ○ Sweats
- ○ Cramping
- ○ Others:_____
- ○ _____

Bowel Movement

BM#1	BM#2	BM#3	BM#4
BM#5	BM#6	BM#7	BM#8

Energy Level   ○ Low   ○ Med   ○ High   **Sleep**
Activity Level ○ Low   ○ Med   ○ High
Mood   ○ Sad   ○ Good ○ Happy   ○ 😐   ○ 🙂

Notes: _____

Date:_____

S M T W T F S

Meals

Exercise:_____

Total Calories Burned:_____

Water Intake

	Time	Food & Drinks	Symptoms	Triggers	Notes
Breakfast					

Carb:_____, Fat:_____, Total Sugar:_____,
Fiber: _____, Protein:_____, Calories:_____

Snack					

Carb:_____, Fat:_____, Total Sugar:_____,
Fiber: _____, Protein:_____, Calories:_____

Lunch					

Carb:_____, Fat:_____, Total Sugar:_____,
Fiber: _____, Protein:_____, Calories:_____

Snack					

Carb:_____, Fat:_____, Total Sugar:_____,
Fiber: _____, Protein:_____, Calories:_____

Dinner					

Carb:_____, Fat:_____, Total Sugar:_____,
Fiber: _____, Protein:_____, Calories:_____

Pain

☹ How severe is the pain?

    1   2   3   4   5

_____
_____

Did you take any medication?_____

Did it help?_____

Where does it hurt?

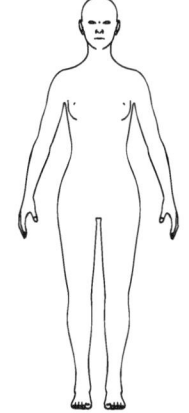

Time	Symptoms	Triggers

Other Symptoms Tracker

- ○ Pain
- ○ Constipation
- ○ Bleeding
- ○ Fatigue
- ○ Bloating
- ○ Sweats
- ○ Cramping
- ○ Others:_____
- ○ _____

Bowel Movement

BM#1	BM#2	BM#3	BM#4
BM#5	BM#6	BM#7	BM#8

Energy Level ○ Low ○ Med ○ High   **Sleep**

Activity Level ○ Low ○ Med ○ High

Mood ○ Sad ○ Good ○ Happy   ○ 😐 ○ 🙂

Notes:

Date:____

S M T W T F S

Meals

Exercise:_____

Total Calories Burned:_____

Water Intake

	Time	Food & Drinks	Symptoms	Triggers	Notes
Breakfast					

Carb:_____, Fat:_____, Total Sugar:_____,
Fiber: _____, Protein:_____, Calories:_____

Snack					

Carb:_____, Fat:_____, Total Sugar:_____,
Fiber: _____, Protein:_____, Calories:_____

Lunch					

Carb:_____, Fat:_____, Total Sugar:_____,
Fiber: _____, Protein:_____, Calories:_____

Snack					

Carb:_____, Fat:_____, Total Sugar:_____,
Fiber: _____, Protein:_____, Calories:_____

Dinner					

Carb:_____, Fat:_____, Total Sugar:_____,
Fiber: _____, Protein:_____, Calories:_____

Pain

Where does it hurt?

How severe is the pain?

1   2   3   4   5

_____
_____

Did you take any medication? _____

Did it help? _____

Time	Symptoms	Triggers

Other Symptoms Tracker

- O Pain
- O Constipation
- O Bleeding
- O Fatigue
- O Bloating
- O Sweats
- O Cramping
- O Others: _____
- O _____

Bowel Movement

BM#1	BM#2	BM#3	BM#4
BM#5	BM#6	BM#7	BM#8

Energy Level   O Low   O Med   O High   **Sleep**
Activity Level O Low   O Med   O High
Mood   O Sad   O Good O Happy   O 😐   O 🙂

Notes: _____

35

Date:_____

S M T W T F S

Meals

Exercise:_____

Total Calories Burned:_____

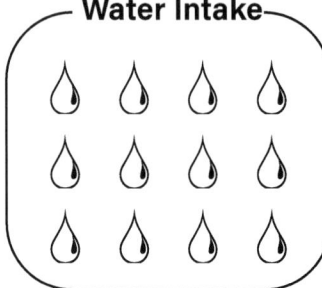
Water Intake

	Time	Food & Drinks	Symptoms	Triggers	Notes
Breakfast					

Carb:_____, Fat:_____, Total Sugar:_____,
Fiber: _____, Protein:_____, Calories:_____

Snack					

Carb:_____, Fat:_____, Total Sugar:_____,
Fiber: _____, Protein:_____, Calories:_____

Lunch					

Carb:_____, Fat:_____, Total Sugar:_____,
Fiber: _____, Protein:_____, Calories:_____

Snack					

Carb:_____, Fat:_____, Total Sugar:_____,
Fiber: _____, Protein:_____, Calories:_____

Dinner					

Carb:_____, Fat:_____, Total Sugar:_____,
Fiber: _____, Protein:_____, Calories:_____

Pain

Where does it hurt?

How severe is the pain?

1   2   3   4   5

_____
_____

Did you take any medication?_____

Did it help?_____

Time	Symptoms	Triggers

Other Symptoms Tracker

- ○ Pain
- ○ Constipation
- ○ Bleeding
- ○ Fatigue
- ○ Bloating
- ○ Sweats
- ○ Cramping
- ○ Others:_____
- ○ _____

Bowel Movement

BM#1	BM#2	BM#3	BM#4
BM#5	BM#6	BM#7	BM#8

Energy Level   ○ Low   ○ Med   ○ High   **Sleep**
Activity Level ○ Low   ○ Med   ○ High
Mood   ○ Sad   ○ Good ○ Happy   ○ 😐   ○ 🙂

Notes: _____

Date:_____

S M T W T F S

Meals

Exercise:_____

Total Calories Burned:_____

Water Intake

	Time	Food & Drinks	Symptoms	Triggers	Notes
Breakfast					

Carb:_____, Fat:_____, Total Sugar:_____,
Fiber: _____, Protein:_____, Calories:_____

Snack					

Carb:_____, Fat:_____, Total Sugar:_____,
Fiber: _____, Protein:_____, Calories:_____

Lunch					

Carb:_____, Fat:_____, Total Sugar:_____,
Fiber: _____, Protein:_____, Calories:_____

Snack					

Carb:_____, Fat:_____, Total Sugar:_____,
Fiber: _____, Protein:_____, Calories:_____

Dinner					

Carb:_____, Fat:_____, Total Sugar:_____,
Fiber: _____, Protein:_____, Calories:_____

Pain

Where does it hurt?

How severe is the pain?

1   2   3   4   5

_____
_____

Did you take any medication? _____

Did it help? _____

Time	Symptoms	Triggers

Other Symptoms Tracker

- ○ Pain
- ○ Constipation
- ○ Bleeding
- ○ Fatigue
- ○ Bloating
- ○ Sweats
- ○ Cramping
- ○ Others:_____
- ○ _____

Bowel Movement

BM#1	BM#2	BM#3	BM#4
BM#5	BM#6	BM#7	BM#8

Energy Level ○ Low ○ Med ○ High

Activity Level ○ Low ○ Med ○ High

Mood ○ Sad ○ Good ○ Happy

Sleep ○ 😐 ○ 🙂

Notes: _____

Date: _____

S M T W T F S

Meals

Exercise: _____

Total Calories Burned: _____

Water Intake

	Time	Food & Drinks	Symptoms	Triggers	Notes
Breakfast					

Carb: _____, Fat: _____, Total Sugar: _____,
Fiber: _____, Protein: _____, Calories: _____

Snack					

Carb: _____, Fat: _____, Total Sugar: _____,
Fiber: _____, Protein: _____, Calories: _____

Lunch					

Carb: _____, Fat: _____, Total Sugar: _____,
Fiber: _____, Protein: _____, Calories: _____

Snack					

Carb: _____, Fat: _____, Total Sugar: _____,
Fiber: _____, Protein: _____, Calories: _____

Dinner					

Carb: _____, Fat: _____, Total Sugar: _____,
Fiber: _____, Protein: _____, Calories: _____

Pain

Where does it hurt?

How severe is the pain?

1 2 3 4 5

_____
_____

Did you take any medication? _____

Did it help? _____

Time	Symptoms	Triggers

Other Symptoms Tracker

- ○ Pain
- ○ Constipation
- ○ Bleeding
- ○ Fatigue
- ○ Bloating
- ○ Sweats
- ○ Cramping
- ○ Others:_____
- ○ _____

Bowel Movement

BM#1	BM#2	BM#3	BM#4
BM#5	BM#6	BM#7	BM#8

Energy Level ○ Low ○ Med ○ High

Activity Level ○ Low ○ Med ○ High

Mood ○ Sad ○ Good ○ Happy

Sleep ○ 😐 ○ 🙂

Notes: _____

Date:_____

S M T W T F S

Meals

Exercise:_____

Total Calories Burned:_____

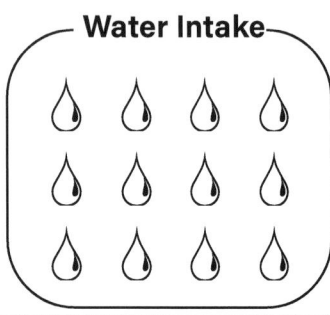
Water Intake

	Time	Food & Drinks	Symptoms	Triggers	Notes
Breakfast					

Carb:_____, Fat:_____, Total Sugar:_____,
Fiber: _____, Protein:_____, Calories:_____

Snack					

Carb:_____, Fat:_____, Total Sugar:_____,
Fiber: _____, Protein:_____, Calories:_____

Lunch					

Carb:_____, Fat:_____, Total Sugar:_____,
Fiber: _____, Protein:_____, Calories:_____

Snack					

Carb:_____, Fat:_____, Total Sugar:_____,
Fiber: _____, Protein:_____, Calories:_____

Dinner					

Carb:_____, Fat:_____, Total Sugar:_____,
Fiber: _____, Protein:_____, Calories:_____

Pain

☹ How severe is the pain? 😮

1   2   3   4   5

_____
_____

Did you take any medication?_____

Did it help?_____

Where does it hurt?

Time	Symptoms	Triggers

Other Symptoms Tracker

- ○ Pain
- ○ Constipation
- ○ Bleeding
- ○ Fatigue
- ○ Bloating
- ○ Sweats
- ○ Cramping
- ○ Others:_____
- ○ _____

Bowel Movement

BM#1	BM#2	BM#3	BM#4
BM#5	BM#6	BM#7	BM#8

Energy Level ○ Low ○ Med ○ High   **Sleep**
Activity Level ○ Low ○ Med ○ High
Mood ○ Sad ○ Good ○ Happy   ○ 😐 ○ 🙂

Notes: _____

Date:_____

S M T W T F S

Meals

Exercise:_____

Total Calories Burned:_____

Water Intake

	Time	Food & Drinks	Symptoms	Triggers	Notes
Breakfast					

Carb:_____, Fat:_____, Total Sugar:_____,
Fiber: _____, Protein:_____, Calories:_____

Snack					

Carb:_____, Fat:_____, Total Sugar:_____,
Fiber: _____, Protein:_____, Calories:_____

Lunch					

Carb:_____, Fat:_____, Total Sugar:_____,
Fiber: _____, Protein:_____, Calories:_____

Snack					

Carb:_____, Fat:_____, Total Sugar:_____,
Fiber: _____, Protein:_____, Calories:_____

Dinner					

Carb:_____, Fat:_____, Total Sugar:_____,
Fiber: _____, Protein:_____, Calories:_____

Pain

Where does it hurt?

How severe is the pain?

1   2   3   4   5

_____
_____

Did you take any medication? _____
Did it help? _____

Time	Symptoms	Triggers

Other Symptoms Tracker

- ○ Pain
- ○ Constipation
- ○ Bleeding
- ○ Fatigue
- ○ Bloating
- ○ Sweats
- ○ Cramping
- ○ Others: _____
- ○ _____

Bowel Movement

BM#1	BM#2	BM#3	BM#4
BM#5	BM#6	BM#7	BM#8

Energy Level   ○ Low   ○ Med   ○ High   **Sleep**
Activity Level   ○ Low   ○ Med   ○ High
Mood   ○ Sad   ○ Good   ○ Happy   ○ 😐   ○ 🙂

Notes: _____

Date:_____

S M T W T F S

Meals

Exercise:_____

Total Calories Burned:_____

Water Intake

	Time	Food & Drinks	Symptoms	Triggers	Notes
Breakfast					

Carb:_____, Fat:_____, Total Sugar:_____,
Fiber: _____, Protein:_____, Calories:_____

Snack					

Carb:_____, Fat:_____, Total Sugar:_____,
Fiber: _____, Protein:_____, Calories:_____

Lunch					

Carb:_____, Fat:_____, Total Sugar:_____,
Fiber: _____, Protein:_____, Calories:_____

Snack					

Carb:_____, Fat:_____, Total Sugar:_____,
Fiber: _____, Protein:_____, Calories:_____

Dinner					

Carb:_____, Fat:_____, Total Sugar:_____,
Fiber: _____, Protein:_____, Calories:_____

Pain

 How severe is the pain?

1   2   3   4   5

_____
_____

Did you take any medication?_____

Did it help?_____

Where does it hurt?

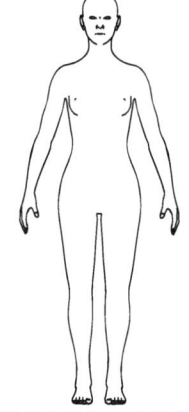

Time	Symptoms	Triggers

Other Symptoms Tracker

- ○ Pain
- ○ Constipation
- ○ Bleeding
- ○ Fatigue
- ○ Bloating
- ○ Sweats
- ○ Cramping
- ○ Others:_____
- ○ _____

Bowel Movement

BM#1	BM#2	BM#3	BM#4
BM#5	BM#6	BM#7	BM#8

Energy Level ○ Low ○ Med ○ High
Activity Level ○ Low ○ Med ○ High
Mood ○ Sad ○ Good ○ Happy

Sleep ○ 😐 ○ 🙂

Notes: _____

Date: _____

S M T W T F S

Meals

Exercise: _____

Total Calories Burned: _____

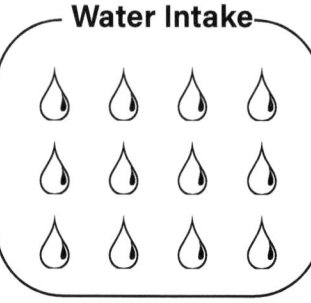
Water Intake

	Time	Food & Drinks	Symptoms	Triggers	Notes
Breakfast					

Carb: _____, Fat: _____, Total Sugar: _____,
Fiber: _____, Protein: _____, Calories: _____

Snack					

Carb: _____, Fat: _____, Total Sugar: _____,
Fiber: _____, Protein: _____, Calories: _____

Lunch					

Carb: _____, Fat: _____, Total Sugar: _____,
Fiber: _____, Protein: _____, Calories: _____

Snack					

Carb: _____, Fat: _____, Total Sugar: _____,
Fiber: _____, Protein: _____, Calories: _____

Dinner					

Carb: _____, Fat: _____, Total Sugar: _____,
Fiber: _____, Protein: _____, Calories: _____

Pain

Where does it hurt?

How severe is the pain?

1   2   3   4   5

_____
_____

Did you take any medication? _____

Did it help? _____

Time	Symptoms	Triggers

Other Symptoms Tracker

- ○ Pain
- ○ Constipation
- ○ Bleeding
- ○ Fatigue
- ○ Bloating
- ○ Sweats
- ○ Cramping
- ○ Others:_____
- ○ _____

Bowel Movement

BM#1	BM#2	BM#3	BM#4
BM#5	BM#6	BM#7	BM#8

Energy Level ○ Low   ○ Med   ○ High

Activity Level ○ Low   ○ Med   ○ High

Mood ○ Sad   ○ Good   ○ Happy

Sleep ○ 😐   ○ 🙂

Notes: _____

Date: _____

S M T W T F S

Meals

Exercise: _____

Total Calories Burned: _____

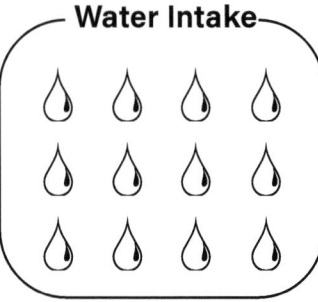
Water Intake

	Time	Food & Drinks	Symptoms	Triggers	Notes
Breakfast					

Carb: _____, Fat: _____, Total Sugar: _____,
Fiber: _____, Protein: _____, Calories: _____

Snack					

Carb: _____, Fat: _____, Total Sugar: _____,
Fiber: _____, Protein: _____, Calories: _____

Lunch					

Carb: _____, Fat: _____, Total Sugar: _____,
Fiber: _____, Protein: _____, Calories: _____

Snack					

Carb: _____, Fat: _____, Total Sugar: _____,
Fiber: _____, Protein: _____, Calories: _____

Dinner					

Carb: _____, Fat: _____, Total Sugar: _____,
Fiber: _____, Protein: _____, Calories: _____

Pain

Where does it hurt?

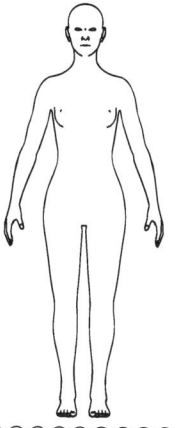

☹ How severe is the pain? 😮

1   2   3   4   5

_____
_____

Did you take any medication? _____

Did it help? _____

Time	Symptoms	Triggers

Other Symptoms Tracker

- ○ Pain
- ○ Constipation
- ○ Bleeding
- ○ Fatigue
- ○ Bloating
- ○ Sweats
- ○ Cramping
- ○ Others:_____
- ○ _____

Bowel Movement

BM#1	BM#2	BM#3	BM#4
BM#5	BM#6	BM#7	BM#8

Energy Level   ○ Low   ○ Med   ○ High   **Sleep**
Activity Level   ○ Low   ○ Med   ○ High
Mood   ○ Sad   ○ Good   ○ Happy   ○ 😐   ○ 🙂

Notes: _____

Date: _____

S M T W T F S

Meals

Exercise: _____

Total Calories Burned: _____

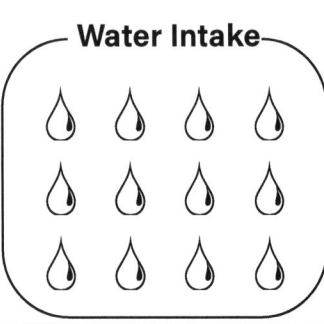
Water Intake

	Time	Food & Drinks	Symptoms	Triggers	Notes
Breakfast					

Carb:_____, Fat:_____, Total Sugar:_____,
Fiber: _____, Protein:_____, Calories:_____

Snack					

Carb:_____, Fat:_____, Total Sugar:_____,
Fiber: _____, Protein:_____, Calories:_____

Lunch					

Carb:_____, Fat:_____, Total Sugar:_____,
Fiber: _____, Protein:_____, Calories:_____

Snack					

Carb:_____, Fat:_____, Total Sugar:_____,
Fiber: _____, Protein:_____, Calories:_____

Dinner					

Carb:_____, Fat:_____, Total Sugar:_____,
Fiber: _____, Protein:_____, Calories:_____

Pain

Where does it hurt?

☹ How severe is the pain? 😮

1   2   3   4   5

_____
_____

Did you take any medication? _____

Did it help? _____

Time	Symptoms	Triggers

Other Symptoms Tracker

- ○ Pain
- ○ Constipation
- ○ Bleeding
- ○ Fatigue
- ○ Bloating
- ○ Sweats
- ○ Cramping
- ○ Others:_____
- ○ _____

Bowel Movement

BM#1	BM#2	BM#3	BM#4
BM#5	BM#6	BM#7	BM#8

Energy Level   ○ Low   ○ Med   ○ High

Activity Level   ○ Low   ○ Med   ○ High

Mood   ○ Sad   ○ Good   ○ Happy

Sleep   ○ 😐   ○ 🙂

Notes: _____

Date: _____

S M T W T F S

Meals

Exercise: _____

Total Calories Burned: _____

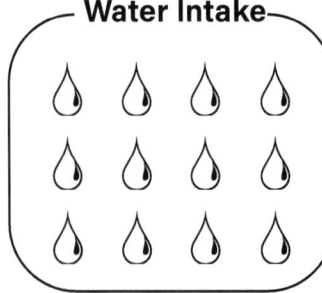
Water Intake

	Time	Food & Drinks	Symptoms	Triggers	Notes
Breakfast					

Carb: _____, Fat: _____, Total Sugar: _____,
Fiber: _____, Protein: _____, Calories: _____

Snack					

Carb: _____, Fat: _____, Total Sugar: _____,
Fiber: _____, Protein: _____, Calories: _____

Lunch					

Carb: _____, Fat: _____, Total Sugar: _____,
Fiber: _____, Protein: _____, Calories: _____

Snack					

Carb: _____, Fat: _____, Total Sugar: _____,
Fiber: _____, Protein: _____, Calories: _____

Dinner					

Carb: _____, Fat: _____, Total Sugar: _____,
Fiber: _____, Protein: _____, Calories: _____

Pain

Where does it hurt?

How severe is the pain?

1 2 3 4 5

_____
_____

Did you take any medication? _____
Did it help? _____

Time	Symptoms	Triggers

Other Symptoms Tracker

- ○ Pain
- ○ Constipation
- ○ Bleeding
- ○ Fatigue
- ○ Bloating
- ○ Sweats
- ○ Cramping
- ○ Others:_____
- ○ _____

Bowel Movement

BM#1	BM#2	BM#3	BM#4
BM#5	BM#6	BM#7	BM#8

Energy Level ○ Low ○ Med ○ High
Activity Level ○ Low ○ Med ○ High
Mood ○ Sad ○ Good ○ Happy

Sleep ○ 😐 ○ 🙂

Notes: _____

Date:_____

S M T W T F S

Meals

Exercise:_____

Total Calories Burned:_____

Water Intake

	Time	Food & Drinks	Symptoms	Triggers	Notes
Breakfast					

Carb:_____, Fat:_____, Total Sugar:_____,
Fiber: _____, Protein:_____, Calories:_____

Snack					

Carb:_____, Fat:_____, Total Sugar:_____,
Fiber: _____, Protein:_____, Calories:_____

Lunch					

Carb:_____, Fat:_____, Total Sugar:_____,
Fiber: _____, Protein:_____, Calories:_____

Snack					

Carb:_____, Fat:_____, Total Sugar:_____,
Fiber: _____, Protein:_____, Calories:_____

Dinner					

Carb:_____, Fat:_____, Total Sugar:_____,
Fiber: _____, Protein:_____, Calories:_____

Pain

Where does it hurt?

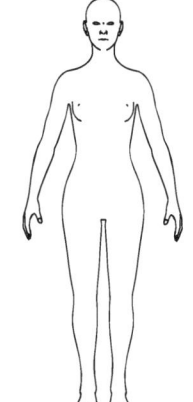

 How severe is the pain?

1 2 3 4 5

_____

_____

Did you take any medication?_____

Did it help?_____

Time	Symptoms	Triggers

Other Symptoms Tracker

- ○ Pain
- ○ Constipation
- ○ Bleeding
- ○ Fatigue
- ○ Bloating
- ○ Sweats
- ○ Cramping
- ○ Others:_____
- ○ _____

Bowel Movement

BM#1	BM#2	BM#3	BM#4
BM#5	BM#6	BM#7	BM#8

Energy Level ○ Low ○ Med ○ High
Activity Level ○ Low ○ Med ○ High
Mood ○ Sad ○ Good ○ Happy

Sleep ○ 😐 ○ ☺

Notes:
_____

Date:_____

S M T W T F S

Meals

Exercise:_____

Total Calories Burned:_____

Water Intake

	Time	Food & Drinks	Symptoms	Triggers	Notes
Breakfast					

Carb:_____, Fat:_____, Total Sugar:_____,
Fiber: _____, Protein:_____, Calories:_____

Snack					

Carb:_____, Fat:_____, Total Sugar:_____,
Fiber: _____, Protein:_____, Calories:_____

Lunch					

Carb:_____, Fat:_____, Total Sugar:_____,
Fiber: _____, Protein:_____, Calories:_____

Snack					

Carb:_____, Fat:_____, Total Sugar:_____,
Fiber: _____, Protein:_____, Calories:_____

Dinner					

Carb:_____, Fat:_____, Total Sugar:_____,
Fiber: _____, Protein:_____, Calories:_____

Pain

Where does it hurt?

 How severe is the pain?

1   2   3   4   5

_____

_____

Did you take any medication?_____

Did it help?_____

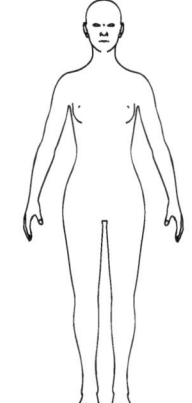

Time	Symptoms	Triggers

Other Symptoms Tracker

- ○ Pain
- ○ Constipation
- ○ Bleeding
- ○ Fatigue
- ○ Bloating
- ○ Sweats
- ○ Cramping
- ○ Others:_____
- ○ _____

Bowel Movement

BM#1	BM#2	BM#3	BM#4
BM#5	BM#6	BM#7	BM#8

Energy Level   ○ Low   ○ Med   ○ High

Activity Level   ○ Low   ○ Med   ○ High

Mood   ○ Sad   ○ Good   ○ Happy

Sleep   ○ 😐   ○ ☺

Notes:
_____

Date:_____

S M T W T F S

Meals

Exercise:_____

Total Calories Burned:_____

Water Intake

	Time	Food & Drinks	Symptoms	Triggers	Notes
Breakfast					

Carb:_____, Fat:_____, Total Sugar:_____,
Fiber: _____, Protein:_____, Calories:_____

	Time	Food & Drinks	Symptoms	Triggers	Notes
Snack					

Carb:_____, Fat:_____, Total Sugar:_____,
Fiber: _____, Protein:_____, Calories:_____

	Time	Food & Drinks	Symptoms	Triggers	Notes
Lunch					

Carb:_____, Fat:_____, Total Sugar:_____,
Fiber: _____, Protein:_____, Calories:_____

	Time	Food & Drinks	Symptoms	Triggers	Notes
Snack					

Carb:_____, Fat:_____, Total Sugar:_____,
Fiber: _____, Protein:_____, Calories:_____

	Time	Food & Drinks	Symptoms	Triggers	Notes
Dinner					

Carb:_____, Fat:_____, Total Sugar:_____,
Fiber: _____, Protein:_____, Calories:_____

Pain

Where does it hurt?

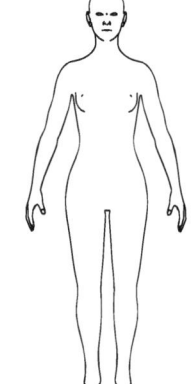

 How severe is the pain? ☺

1   2   3   4   5

_____

_____

Did you take any medication?_____

Did it help?_____

Time	Symptoms	Triggers

Other Symptoms Tracker

- ○ Pain
- ○ Constipation
- ○ Bleeding
- ○ Fatigue
- ○ Bloating
- ○ Sweats
- ○ Cramping
- ○ Others:_____
- ○ _____

Bowel Movement

BM#1	BM#2	BM#3	BM#4
BM#5	BM#6	BM#7	BM#8

Energy Level ○ Low   ○ Med   ○ High

Activity Level ○ Low   ○ Med   ○ High

Mood ○ Sad   ○ Good   ○ Happy

Sleep ○ 😐   ○ 🙂

Notes:
_____

$\mathcal{D}ate:$ _____

S M T W T F S

Meals

Exercise: _____

Total Calories Burned: _____

Water Intake

	Time	Food & Drinks	Symptoms	Triggers	Notes
Breakfast					

Carb: _____, Fat: _____, Total Sugar: _____,
Fiber: _____, Protein: _____, Calories: _____

	Time	Food & Drinks	Symptoms	Triggers	Notes
Snack					

Carb: _____, Fat: _____, Total Sugar: _____,
Fiber: _____, Protein: _____, Calories: _____

	Time	Food & Drinks	Symptoms	Triggers	Notes
Lunch					

Carb: _____, Fat: _____, Total Sugar: _____,
Fiber: _____, Protein: _____, Calories: _____

	Time	Food & Drinks	Symptoms	Triggers	Notes
Snack					

Carb: _____, Fat: _____, Total Sugar: _____,
Fiber: _____, Protein: _____, Calories: _____

	Time	Food & Drinks	Symptoms	Triggers	Notes
Dinner					

Carb: _____, Fat: _____, Total Sugar: _____,
Fiber: _____, Protein: _____, Calories: _____

Pain

😣 How severe is the pain? 😮

1   2   3   4   5

_____

_____

Did you take any medication?_____

Did it help?_____

Where does it hurt?

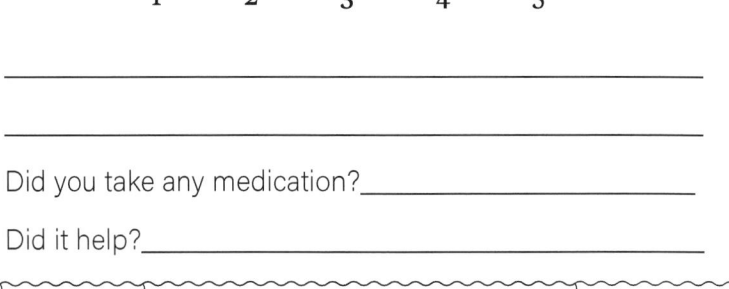

Time	Symptoms	Triggers

Other Symptoms Tracker

- ○ Pain
- ○ Constipation
- ○ Bleeding
- ○ Fatigue
- ○ Bloating
- ○ Sweats
- ○ Cramping
- ○ Others:_____
- ○ _____

Bowel Movement

BM#1	BM#2	BM#3	BM#4
BM#5	BM#6	BM#7	BM#8

Energy Level   ○ Low   ○ Med   ○ High
Activity Level ○ Low   ○ Med   ○ High
Mood   ○ Sad   ○ Good ○ Happy

Sleep ○ 😐 ○ 🙂

Notes:
_____

63

Date:_____

S M T W T F S

Meals

Exercise:_____

Total Calories Burned:_____

Water Intake

	Time	Food & Drinks	Symptoms	Triggers	Notes
Breakfast					

Carb:_____, Fat:_____, Total Sugar:_____,
Fiber: _____, Protein:_____, Calories:_____

Snack					

Carb:_____, Fat:_____, Total Sugar:_____,
Fiber: _____, Protein:_____, Calories:_____

Lunch					

Carb:_____, Fat:_____, Total Sugar:_____,
Fiber: _____, Protein:_____, Calories:_____

Snack					

Carb:_____, Fat:_____, Total Sugar:_____,
Fiber: _____, Protein:_____, Calories:_____

Dinner					

Carb:_____, Fat:_____, Total Sugar:_____,
Fiber: _____, Protein:_____, Calories:_____

Pain

 How severe is the pain? 😮

1   2   3   4   5

_____
_____

Did you take any medication? _____

Did it help? _____

Where does it hurt?

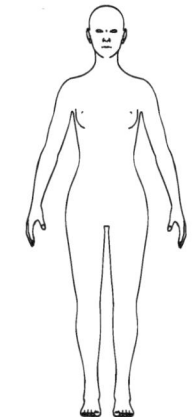

Time	Symptoms	Triggers

Other Symptoms Tracker

- ◯ Pain
- ◯ Constipation
- ◯ Bleeding
- ◯ Fatigue
- ◯ Bloating
- ◯ Sweats
- ◯ Cramping
- ◯ Others: _____
- ◯ _____

Bowel Movement

BM#1	BM#2	BM#3	BM#4
BM#5	BM#6	BM#7	BM#8

Energy Level ◯ Low ◯ Med ◯ High

Activity Level ◯ Low ◯ Med ◯ High

Mood ◯ Sad ◯ Good ◯ Happy

Sleep ◯ 😐 ◯ 🙂

Notes: _____

Date: _____

S M T W T F S

Meals

Exercise: _____

Total Calories Burned: _____

Water Intake

	Time	Food & Drinks	Symptoms	Triggers	Notes
Breakfast					

Carb: _____, Fat: _____, Total Sugar: _____,
Fiber: _____, Protein: _____, Calories: _____

Snack					

Carb: _____, Fat: _____, Total Sugar: _____,
Fiber: _____, Protein: _____, Calories: _____

Lunch					

Carb: _____, Fat: _____, Total Sugar: _____,
Fiber: _____, Protein: _____, Calories: _____

Snack					

Carb: _____, Fat: _____, Total Sugar: _____,
Fiber: _____, Protein: _____, Calories: _____

Dinner					

Carb: _____, Fat: _____, Total Sugar: _____,
Fiber: _____, Protein: _____, Calories: _____

Pain

Where does it hurt?

How severe is the pain?

1   2   3   4   5

_____
_____

Did you take any medication?_____

Did it help?_____

Time	Symptoms	Triggers

Other Symptoms Tracker

- ○ Pain
- ○ Constipation
- ○ Bleeding
- ○ Fatigue
- ○ Bloating
- ○ Sweats
- ○ Cramping
- ○ Others:_____
- ○ _____

Bowel Movement

BM#1	BM#2	BM#3	BM#4
BM#5	BM#6	BM#7	BM#8

Energy Level   ○ Low   ○ Med   ○ High
Activity Level   ○ Low   ○ Med   ○ High
Mood   ○ Sad   ○ Good   ○ Happy

Sleep   ○ 😐   ○ ☺

Notes:
_____

Date: _____

S M T W T F S

Meals

Exercise: _____

Total Calories Burned: _____

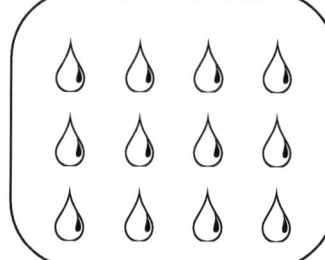
Water Intake

	Time	Food & Drinks	Symptoms	Triggers	Notes
Breakfast					

Carb: _____, Fat: _____, Total Sugar: _____,
Fiber: _____, Protein: _____, Calories: _____

Snack					

Carb: _____, Fat: _____, Total Sugar: _____,
Fiber: _____, Protein: _____, Calories: _____

Lunch					

Carb: _____, Fat: _____, Total Sugar: _____,
Fiber: _____, Protein: _____, Calories: _____

Snack					

Carb: _____, Fat: _____, Total Sugar: _____,
Fiber: _____, Protein: _____, Calories: _____

Dinner					

Carb: _____, Fat: _____, Total Sugar: _____,
Fiber: _____, Protein: _____, Calories: _____

Pain

Where does it hurt?

How severe is the pain?

1   2   3   4   5

_____
_____

Did you take any medication?_____
Did it help?_____

Time	Symptoms	Triggers

Other Symptoms Tracker

- ○ Pain
- ○ Constipation
- ○ Bleeding
- ○ Fatigue
- ○ Bloating
- ○ Sweats
- ○ Cramping
- ○ Others:_____
- ○ _____

Bowel Movement

BM#1	BM#2	BM#3	BM#4
BM#5	BM#6	BM#7	BM#8

Energy Level   ○ Low   ○ Med   ○ High
Activity Level ○ Low   ○ Med   ○ High
Mood   ○ Sad   ○ Good ○ Happy

Sleep   ○ 😐   ○ ☺

Notes: _____

Date: _____

S M T W T F S

Meals

Exercise: _____

Total Calories Burned: _____

Water Intake

	Time	Food & Drinks	Symptoms	Triggers	Notes
Breakfast					

Carb: _____, Fat: _____, Total Sugar: _____,
Fiber: _____, Protein: _____, Calories: _____

Snack					

Carb: _____, Fat: _____, Total Sugar: _____,
Fiber: _____, Protein: _____, Calories: _____

Lunch					

Carb: _____, Fat: _____, Total Sugar: _____,
Fiber: _____, Protein: _____, Calories: _____

Snack					

Carb: _____, Fat: _____, Total Sugar: _____,
Fiber: _____, Protein: _____, Calories: _____

Dinner					

Carb: _____, Fat: _____, Total Sugar: _____,
Fiber: _____, Protein: _____, Calories: _____

Pain

Where does it hurt?

How severe is the pain?

1   2   3   4   5

_____

_____

Did you take any medication?_____

Did it help?_____

Time	Symptoms	Triggers

Other Symptoms Tracker

- ○ Pain
- ○ Constipation
- ○ Bleeding
- ○ Fatigue
- ○ Bloating
- ○ Sweats
- ○ Cramping
- ○ Others:_____
- ○ _____

Bowel Movement

BM#1	BM#2	BM#3	BM#4
BM#5	BM#6	BM#7	BM#8

Energy Level	○ Low	○ Med	○ High	**Sleep**
Activity Level	○ Low	○ Med	○ High	
Mood	○ Sad	○ Good	○ Happy	○ 😐 ○ 🙂

Notes:
_____

Date:_____

S M T W T F S

Meals

Exercise:_____

Total Calories Burned:_____

Water Intake

	Time	Food & Drinks	Symptoms	Triggers	Notes
Breakfast					

Carb:_____, Fat:_____, Total Sugar:_____,
Fiber: _____, Protein:_____, Calories:_____

Snack					

Carb:_____, Fat:_____, Total Sugar:_____,
Fiber: _____, Protein:_____, Calories:_____

Lunch					

Carb:_____, Fat:_____, Total Sugar:_____,
Fiber: _____, Protein:_____, Calories:_____

Snack					

Carb:_____, Fat:_____, Total Sugar:_____,
Fiber: _____, Protein:_____, Calories:_____

Dinner					

Carb:_____, Fat:_____, Total Sugar:_____,
Fiber: _____, Protein:_____, Calories:_____

Pain

Where does it hurt?

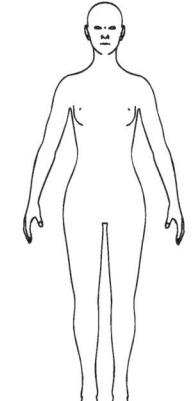

 How severe is the pain?

1 2 3 4 5

_____
_____

Did you take any medication? _____

Did it help? _____

Time	Symptoms	Triggers

Other Symptoms Tracker

- O Pain
- O Constipation
- O Bleeding
- O Fatigue
- O Bloating
- O Sweats
- O Cramping
- O Others: _____
- O _____

Bowel Movement

BM#1	BM#2	BM#3	BM#4
BM#5	BM#6	BM#7	BM#8

Energy Level   O Low   O Med   O High   **Sleep**
Activity Level O Low   O Med   O High
Mood   O Sad   O Good O Happy

Notes:
_____

Date:_____

S M T W T F S

Meals

Exercise:_____

Total Calories Burned:_____

Water Intake

	Time	Food & Drinks	Symptoms	Triggers	Notes
Breakfast					

Carb:_____, Fat:_____, Total Sugar:_____,
Fiber: _____, Protein:_____, Calories:_____

	Time	Food & Drinks	Symptoms	Triggers	Notes
Snack					

Carb:_____, Fat:_____, Total Sugar:_____,
Fiber: _____, Protein:_____, Calories:_____

	Time	Food & Drinks	Symptoms	Triggers	Notes
Lunch					

Carb:_____, Fat:_____, Total Sugar:_____,
Fiber: _____, Protein:_____, Calories:_____

	Time	Food & Drinks	Symptoms	Triggers	Notes
Snack					

Carb:_____, Fat:_____, Total Sugar:_____,
Fiber: _____, Protein:_____, Calories:_____

	Time	Food & Drinks	Symptoms	Triggers	Notes
Dinner					

Carb:_____, Fat:_____, Total Sugar:_____,
Fiber: _____, Protein:_____, Calories:_____

Pain

Where does it hurt?

☹ How severe is the pain? 😊

1   2   3   4   5

_____
_____

Did you take any medication?_____

Did it help?_____

Time	Symptoms	Triggers

Other Symptoms Tracker

- ○ Pain
- ○ Constipation
- ○ Bleeding
- ○ Fatigue
- ○ Bloating
- ○ Sweats
- ○ Cramping
- ○ Others:_____
- ○ _____

Bowel Movement

BM#1	BM#2	BM#3	BM#4
BM#5	BM#6	BM#7	BM#8

Energy Level   ○ Low   ○ Med   ○ High
Activity Level   ○ Low   ○ Med   ○ High
Mood   ○ Sad   ○ Good   ○ Happy

Sleep   ○ 😐   ○ 🙂

Notes:
_____

Date: _____

S M T W T F S

Meals

Exercise: _____

Total Calories Burned: _____

Water Intake

	Time	Food & Drinks	Symptoms	Triggers	Notes
Breakfast					

Carb: _____, Fat: _____, Total Sugar: _____,
Fiber: _____, Protein: _____, Calories: _____

Snack					

Carb: _____, Fat: _____, Total Sugar: _____,
Fiber: _____, Protein: _____, Calories: _____

Lunch					

Carb: _____, Fat: _____, Total Sugar: _____,
Fiber: _____, Protein: _____, Calories: _____

Snack					

Carb: _____, Fat: _____, Total Sugar: _____,
Fiber: _____, Protein: _____, Calories: _____

Dinner					

Carb: _____, Fat: _____, Total Sugar: _____,
Fiber: _____, Protein: _____, Calories: _____

Pain

Where does it hurt?

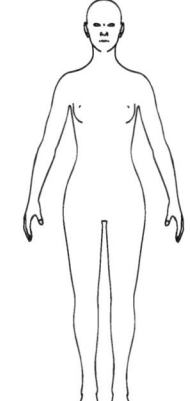

 How severe is the pain?

1   2   3   4   5

_____
_____

Did you take any medication?_____

Did it help?_____

Time	Symptoms	Triggers

Other Symptoms Tracker

- ○ Pain
- ○ Constipation
- ○ Bleeding
- ○ Fatigue
- ○ Bloating
- ○ Sweats
- ○ Cramping
- ○ Others:_____
- ○ _____

Bowel Movement

BM#1	BM#2	BM#3	BM#4
BM#5	BM#6	BM#7	BM#8

Energy Level ○ Low   ○ Med   ○ High
Activity Level ○ Low   ○ Med   ○ High
Mood ○ Sad   ○ Good   ○ Happy

Sleep ○ 😐   ○ 🙂

Notes:
_____

Date:_____

S M T W T F S

Meals

Exercise:_____

Total Calories Burned:_____

Water Intake

	Time	Food & Drinks	Symptoms	Triggers	Notes
Breakfast					

Carb:_____, Fat:_____, Total Sugar:_____,
Fiber: _____, Protein:_____, Calories:_____

Snack					

Carb:_____, Fat:_____, Total Sugar:_____,
Fiber: _____, Protein:_____, Calories:_____

Lunch					

Carb:_____, Fat:_____, Total Sugar:_____,
Fiber: _____, Protein:_____, Calories:_____

Snack					

Carb:_____, Fat:_____, Total Sugar:_____,
Fiber: _____, Protein:_____, Calories:_____

Dinner					

Carb:_____, Fat:_____, Total Sugar:_____,
Fiber: _____, Protein:_____, Calories:_____

Pain

Where does it hurt?

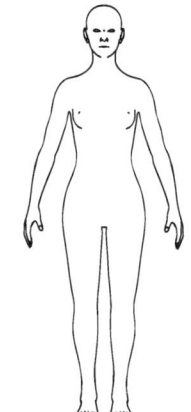

 How severe is the pain?

   1   2   3   4   5

_____

_____

Did you take any medication?_____

Did it help?_____

Time	Symptoms	Triggers

Other Symptoms Tracker

- ○ Pain
- ○ Constipation
- ○ Bleeding
- ○ Fatigue
- ○ Bloating
- ○ Sweats
- ○ Cramping
- ○ Others:_____
- ○ _____

Bowel Movement

BM#1	BM#2	BM#3	BM#4
BM#5	BM#6	BM#7	BM#8

Energy Level   ○ Low   ○ Med   ○ High
Activity Level   ○ Low   ○ Med   ○ High
Mood   ○ Sad   ○ Good   ○ Happy

Sleep   ○ 😐   ○ 🙂

Notes:
_____

Date:_____

S M T W T F S

Meals

Exercise:_____

Total Calories Burned:_____

Water Intake

	Time	Food & Drinks	Symptoms	Triggers	Notes
Breakfast					

Carb:_____, Fat:_____, Total Sugar:_____,
Fiber: _____, Protein:_____, Calories:_____

Snack					

Carb:_____, Fat:_____, Total Sugar:_____,
Fiber: _____, Protein:_____, Calories:_____

Lunch					

Carb:_____, Fat:_____, Total Sugar:_____,
Fiber: _____, Protein:_____, Calories:_____

Snack					

Carb:_____, Fat:_____, Total Sugar:_____,
Fiber: _____, Protein:_____, Calories:_____

Dinner					

Carb:_____, Fat:_____, Total Sugar:_____,
Fiber: _____, Protein:_____, Calories:_____

Pain

Where does it hurt?

 How severe is the pain?

1   2   3   4   5

_____

_____

Did you take any medication?_____

Did it help?_____

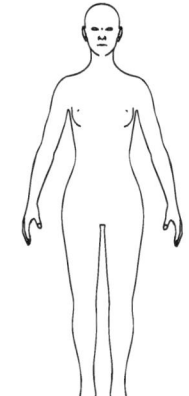

Time	Symptoms	Triggers

Other Symptoms Tracker

- ○ Pain
- ○ Constipation
- ○ Bleeding
- ○ Fatigue
- ○ Bloating
- ○ Sweats
- ○ Cramping
- ○ Others:_____
- ○ _____

Bowel Movement

BM#1	BM#2	BM#3	BM#4
BM#5	BM#6	BM#7	BM#8

Energy Level ○ Low ○ Med ○ High
Activity Level ○ Low ○ Med ○ High
Mood ○ Sad ○ Good ○ Happy

Sleep ○ 😐 ○ 🙂

Notes:
_____

Date:_____

S M T W T F S

Meals

Exercise:_____

Total Calories Burned:_____

Water Intake

	Time	Food & Drinks	Symptoms	Triggers	Notes
Breakfast					

Carb:_____, Fat:_____, Total Sugar:_____,
Fiber: _____, Protein:_____, Calories:_____

Snack					

Carb:_____, Fat:_____, Total Sugar:_____,
Fiber: _____, Protein:_____, Calories:_____

Lunch					

Carb:_____, Fat:_____, Total Sugar:_____,
Fiber: _____, Protein:_____, Calories:_____

Snack					

Carb:_____, Fat:_____, Total Sugar:_____,
Fiber: _____, Protein:_____, Calories:_____

Dinner					

Carb:_____, Fat:_____, Total Sugar:_____,
Fiber: _____, Protein:_____, Calories:_____

Pain

Where does it hurt?

 How severe is the pain?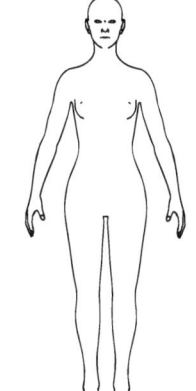

1   2   3   4   5

_____
_____

Did you take any medication?_____

Did it help?_____

Time	Symptoms	Triggers

Other Symptoms Tracker

- O Pain
- O Constipation
- O Bleeding
- O Fatigue
- O Bloating
- O Sweats
- O Cramping
- O Others:_____
- O _____

Bowel Movement

BM#1	BM#2	BM#3	BM#4
BM#5	BM#6	BM#7	BM#8

Energy Level   O Low   O Med   O High   **Sleep**
Activity Level   O Low   O Med   O High
Mood   O Sad   O Good   O Happy   O 😐   O 🙂

Notes:
_____

Date:_____

S M T W T F S

Meals

Exercise:_____

Total Calories Burned:_____

Water Intake

	Time	Food & Drinks	Symptoms	Triggers	Notes
Breakfast					

Carb:_____, Fat:_____, Total Sugar:_____,
Fiber: _____, Protein:_____, Calories:_____

Snack					

Carb:_____, Fat:_____, Total Sugar:_____,
Fiber: _____, Protein:_____, Calories:_____

Lunch					

Carb:_____, Fat:_____, Total Sugar:_____,
Fiber: _____, Protein:_____, Calories:_____

Snack					

Carb:_____, Fat:_____, Total Sugar:_____,
Fiber: _____, Protein:_____, Calories:_____

Dinner					

Carb:_____, Fat:_____, Total Sugar:_____,
Fiber: _____, Protein:_____, Calories:_____

Pain

Where does it hurt?

 How severe is the pain?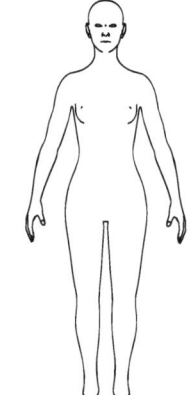

1   2   3   4   5

_____

_____

Did you take any medication?_____

Did it help?_____

Time	Symptoms	Triggers

Other Symptoms Tracker

- O Pain
- O Constipation
- O Bleeding
- O Fatigue
- O Bloating
- O Sweats
- O Cramping
- O Others:_____
- O _____

Bowel Movement

BM#1	BM#2	BM#3	BM#4
BM#5	BM#6	BM#7	BM#8

Energy Level   O Low   O Med   O High   **Sleep**
Activity Level O Low   O Med   O High
Mood   O Sad   O Good O Happy   O 😐   O 🙂

Notes:
_____

Date:_____

S M T W T F S

Meals

Exercise:_____

Total Calories Burned:_____

Water Intake

	Time	Food & Drinks	Symptoms	Triggers	Notes
Breakfast					

Carb:_____, Fat:_____, Total Sugar:_____,
Fiber: _____, Protein:_____, Calories:_____

Snack					

Carb:_____, Fat:_____, Total Sugar:_____,
Fiber: _____, Protein:_____, Calories:_____

Lunch					

Carb:_____, Fat:_____, Total Sugar:_____,
Fiber: _____, Protein:_____, Calories:_____

Snack					

Carb:_____, Fat:_____, Total Sugar:_____,
Fiber: _____, Protein:_____, Calories:_____

Dinner					

Carb:_____, Fat:_____, Total Sugar:_____,
Fiber: _____, Protein:_____, Calories:_____

Pain

 How severe is the pain?

1   2   3   4   5

_____

_____

Did you take any medication?_____

Did it help?_____

Where does it hurt?

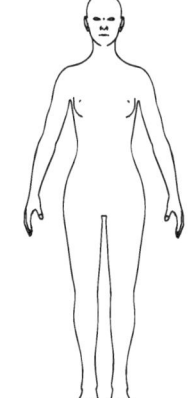

Time	Symptoms	Triggers

Other Symptoms Tracker

- ○ Pain
- ○ Constipation
- ○ Bleeding
- ○ Fatigue
- ○ Bloating
- ○ Sweats
- ○ Cramping
- ○ Others:_____
- ○ _____

Bowel Movement

BM#1	BM#2	BM#3	BM#4
BM#5	BM#6	BM#7	BM#8

Energy Level   ○ Low   ○ Med   ○ High
Activity Level   ○ Low   ○ Med   ○ High
Mood   ○ Sad   ○ Good   ○ Happy

Sleep   ○   ○

Notes:
_____

Date:_____

S M T W T F S

Meals

Exercise:_____

Total Calories Burned:_____

Water Intake

	Time	Food & Drinks	Symptoms	Triggers	Notes
Breakfast					

Carb:_____, Fat:_____, Total Sugar:_____,
Fiber: _____, Protein:_____, Calories:_____

Snack					

Carb:_____, Fat:_____, Total Sugar:_____,
Fiber: _____, Protein:_____, Calories:_____

Lunch					

Carb:_____, Fat:_____, Total Sugar:_____,
Fiber: _____, Protein:_____, Calories:_____

Snack					

Carb:_____, Fat:_____, Total Sugar:_____,
Fiber: _____, Protein:_____, Calories:_____

Dinner					

Carb:_____, Fat:_____, Total Sugar:_____,
Fiber: _____, Protein:_____, Calories:_____

Pain

Where does it hurt?

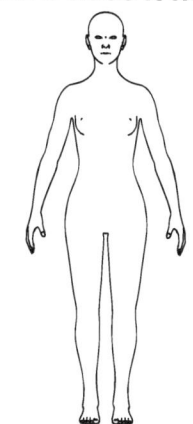

How severe is the pain?

1   2   3   4   5

_____

_____

Did you take any medication?_____

Did it help?_____

Time	Symptoms	Triggers

Other Symptoms Tracker

- ○ Pain
- ○ Constipation
- ○ Bleeding
- ○ Fatigue
- ○ Bloating
- ○ Sweats
- ○ Cramping
- ○ Others:_____
- ○ _____

Bowel Movement

BM#1	BM#2	BM#3	BM#4
BM#5	BM#6	BM#7	BM#8

Energy Level   ○ Low   ○ Med   ○ High

Activity Level   ○ Low   ○ Med   ○ High

Mood   ○ Sad   ○ Good   ○ Happy

Sleep

Notes:
_____

Date:_____

S M T W T F S

Meals

Exercise:_____

Total Calories Burned:_____

Water Intake

	Time	Food & Drinks	Symptoms	Triggers	Notes
Breakfast					

Carb:_____, Fat:_____, Total Sugar:_____,
Fiber: _____, Protein:_____, Calories:_____

Snack					

Carb:_____, Fat:_____, Total Sugar:_____,
Fiber: _____, Protein:_____, Calories:_____

Lunch					

Carb:_____, Fat:_____, Total Sugar:_____,
Fiber: _____, Protein:_____, Calories:_____

Snack					

Carb:_____, Fat:_____, Total Sugar:_____,
Fiber: _____, Protein:_____, Calories:_____

Dinner					

Carb:_____, Fat:_____, Total Sugar:_____,
Fiber: _____, Protein:_____, Calories:_____

Pain

Where does it hurt?

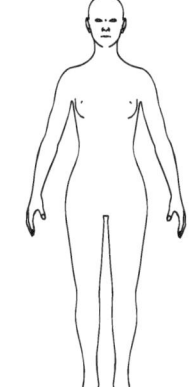

 How severe is the pain?

1 2 3 4 5

_____
_____

Did you take any medication?_____

Did it help?_____

Time	Symptoms	Triggers

Other Symptoms Tracker

- ○ Pain
- ○ Constipation
- ○ Bleeding
- ○ Fatigue
- ○ Bloating
- ○ Sweats
- ○ Cramping
- ○ Others:_____
- ○ _____

Bowel Movement

BM#1	BM#2	BM#3	BM#4
BM#5	BM#6	BM#7	BM#8

Energy Level ○ Low ○ Med ○ High
Activity Level ○ Low ○ Med ○ High
Mood ○ Sad ○ Good ○ Happy

Sleep ○ 😐 ○ 🙂

Notes:
_____

Date:_____

S M T W T F S

Meals

Exercise:_____

Total Calories Burned:_____

Water Intake

	Time	Food & Drinks	Symptoms	Triggers	Notes
Breakfast					

Carb:_____, Fat:_____, Total Sugar:_____,
Fiber: _____, Protein:_____, Calories:_____

Snack					

Carb:_____, Fat:_____, Total Sugar:_____,
Fiber: _____, Protein:_____, Calories:_____

Lunch					

Carb:_____, Fat:_____, Total Sugar:_____,
Fiber: _____, Protein:_____, Calories:_____

Snack					

Carb:_____, Fat:_____, Total Sugar:_____,
Fiber: _____, Protein:_____, Calories:_____

Dinner					

Carb:_____, Fat:_____, Total Sugar:_____,
Fiber: _____, Protein:_____, Calories:_____

Pain

Where does it hurt?

 How severe is the pain?

1   2   3   4   5

_____
_____

Did you take any medication?_____

Did it help?_____

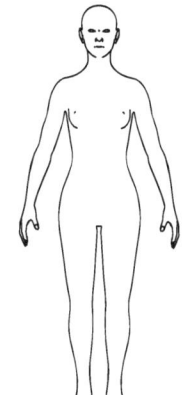

Time	Symptoms	Triggers

Other Symptoms Tracker

- O Pain
- O Constipation
- O Bleeding
- O Fatigue
- O Bloating
- O Sweats
- O Cramping
- O Others:_____
- O _____

Bowel Movement

BM#1	BM#2	BM#3	BM#4
BM#5	BM#6	BM#7	BM#8

Energy Level   O Low   O Med   O High   **Sleep**
Activity Level   O Low   O Med   O High
Mood   O Sad   O Good   O Happy   O   O

Notes:
_____

Date:_____

S M T W T F S

Meals

Exercise:_____

Total Calories Burned:_____

Water Intake

	Time	Food & Drinks	Symptoms	Triggers	Notes
Breakfast					

Carb:_____, Fat:_____, Total Sugar:_____,
Fiber: _____, Protein:_____, Calories:_____

Snack					

Carb:_____, Fat:_____, Total Sugar:_____,
Fiber: _____, Protein:_____, Calories:_____

Lunch					

Carb:_____, Fat:_____, Total Sugar:_____,
Fiber: _____, Protein:_____, Calories:_____

Snack					

Carb:_____, Fat:_____, Total Sugar:_____,
Fiber: _____, Protein:_____, Calories:_____

Dinner					

Carb:_____, Fat:_____, Total Sugar:_____,
Fiber: _____, Protein:_____, Calories:_____

Pain

Where does it hurt?

☹ How severe is the pain? 😣

1   2   3   4   5

_____
_____

Did you take any medication? _____

Did it help? _____

Time	Symptoms	Triggers

Other Symptoms Tracker

- ○ Pain
- ○ Constipation
- ○ Bleeding
- ○ Fatigue
- ○ Bloating
- ○ Sweats
- ○ Cramping
- ○ Others: _____
- ○ _____

Bowel Movement

BM#1	BM#2	BM#3	BM#4
BM#5	BM#6	BM#7	BM#8

Energy Level   ○ Low   ○ Med   ○ High

Activity Level   ○ Low   ○ Med   ○ High

Mood   ○ Sad   ○ Good   ○ Happy

Sleep   ○ 😐   ○ 🙂

Notes:
_____

Date: _____

S M T W T F S

Meals

Exercise: _____

Total Calories Burned: _____

Water Intake

	Time	Food & Drinks	Symptoms	Triggers	Notes
Breakfast					

Carb: _____, Fat: _____, Total Sugar: _____,
Fiber: _____, Protein: _____, Calories: _____

Snack					

Carb: _____, Fat: _____, Total Sugar: _____,
Fiber: _____, Protein: _____, Calories: _____

Lunch					

Carb: _____, Fat: _____, Total Sugar: _____,
Fiber: _____, Protein: _____, Calories: _____

Snack					

Carb: _____, Fat: _____, Total Sugar: _____,
Fiber: _____, Protein: _____, Calories: _____

Dinner					

Carb: _____, Fat: _____, Total Sugar: _____,
Fiber: _____, Protein: _____, Calories: _____

Pain

 How severe is the pain?

1   2   3   4   5

_____
_____

Did you take any medication?_____
Did it help?_____

Where does it hurt?

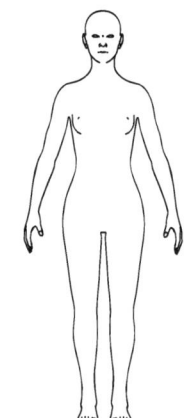

Time	Symptoms	Triggers

Other Symptoms Tracker

- O Pain
- O Constipation
- O Bleeding
- O Fatigue
- O Bloating
- O Sweats
- O Cramping
- O Others:_____
- O _____

Bowel Movement

BM#1	BM#2	BM#3	BM#4
BM#5	BM#6	BM#7	BM#8

Energy Level O Low   O Med   O High
Activity Level O Low   O Med   O High
Mood   O Sad   O Good O Happy

Sleep

Notes: _____

Date: _____

S M T W T F S

Meals

Exercise: _____

Total Calories Burned: _____

Water Intake

	Time	Food & Drinks	Symptoms	Triggers	Notes
Breakfast					

Carb:_____, Fat:_____, Total Sugar:_____,
Fiber: _____, Protein:_____, Calories:_____

	Time	Food & Drinks	Symptoms	Triggers	Notes
Snack					

Carb:_____, Fat:_____, Total Sugar:_____,
Fiber: _____, Protein:_____, Calories:_____

	Time	Food & Drinks	Symptoms	Triggers	Notes
Lunch					

Carb:_____, Fat:_____, Total Sugar:_____,
Fiber: _____, Protein:_____, Calories:_____

	Time	Food & Drinks	Symptoms	Triggers	Notes
Snack					

Carb:_____, Fat:_____, Total Sugar:_____,
Fiber: _____, Protein:_____, Calories:_____

	Time	Food & Drinks	Symptoms	Triggers	Notes
Dinner					

Carb:_____, Fat:_____, Total Sugar:_____,
Fiber: _____, Protein:_____, Calories:_____

Pain

Where does it hurt?

☹ How severe is the pain? 😵

1   2   3   4   5

_____

_____

Did you take any medication?_____

Did it help?_____

Time	Symptoms	Triggers

Other Symptoms Tracker

- ○ Pain
- ○ Constipation
- ○ Bleeding
- ○ Fatigue
- ○ Bloating
- ○ Sweats
- ○ Cramping
- ○ Others:_____
- ○ _____

Bowel Movement

BM#1	BM#2	BM#3	BM#4
BM#5	BM#6	BM#7	BM#8

Energy Level   ○ Low   ○ Med   ○ High
Activity Level ○ Low   ○ Med   ○ High
Mood   ○ Sad   ○ Good ○ Happy

Sleep   ○ 😐   ○ 🙂

Notes: _____

Date:_____

S M T W T F S

Meals

Exercise:_____

Total Calories Burned:_____

Water Intake

	Time	Food & Drinks	Symptoms	Triggers	Notes
Breakfast					

Carb:_____, Fat:_____, Total Sugar:_____,
Fiber: _____, Protein:_____, Calories:_____

Snack					

Carb:_____, Fat:_____, Total Sugar:_____,
Fiber: _____, Protein:_____, Calories:_____

Lunch					

Carb:_____, Fat:_____, Total Sugar:_____,
Fiber: _____, Protein:_____, Calories:_____

Snack					

Carb:_____, Fat:_____, Total Sugar:_____,
Fiber: _____, Protein:_____, Calories:_____

Dinner					

Carb:_____, Fat:_____, Total Sugar:_____,
Fiber: _____, Protein:_____, Calories:_____

Pain

How severe is the pain?

1   2   3   4   5

_____
_____

Did you take any medication? _____

Did it help? _____

Where does it hurt?

Time	Symptoms	Triggers

Other Symptoms Tracker

- ○ Pain
- ○ Constipation
- ○ Bleeding
- ○ Fatigue
- ○ Bloating
- ○ Sweats
- ○ Cramping
- ○ Others: _____
- ○ _____

Bowel Movement

BM#1	BM#2	BM#3	BM#4
BM#5	BM#6	BM#7	BM#8

Energy Level   ○ Low   ○ Med   ○ High

Activity Level   ○ Low   ○ Med   ○ High

Mood   ○ Sad   ○ Good   ○ Happy

Sleep   ○ 😐   ○ 🙂

Notes: _____

Date:_____

S M T W T F S

Meals

Exercise:_____

Total Calories Burned:_____

Water Intake

	Time	Food & Drinks	Symptoms	Triggers	Notes
Breakfast					

Carb:_____, Fat:_____, Total Sugar:_____,
Fiber: _____, Protein:_____, Calories:_____

Snack					

Carb:_____, Fat:_____, Total Sugar:_____,
Fiber: _____, Protein:_____, Calories:_____

Lunch					

Carb:_____, Fat:_____, Total Sugar:_____,
Fiber: _____, Protein:_____, Calories:_____

Snack					

Carb:_____, Fat:_____, Total Sugar:_____,
Fiber: _____, Protein:_____, Calories:_____

Dinner					

Carb:_____, Fat:_____, Total Sugar:_____,
Fiber: _____, Protein:_____, Calories:_____

Pain

☹ How severe is the pain? 😵

1 2 3 4 5

_____
_____

Did you take any medication? _____

Did it help? _____

Where does it hurt?

Time	Symptoms	Triggers

Other Symptoms Tracker

- ○ Pain
- ○ Constipation
- ○ Bleeding
- ○ Fatigue
- ○ Bloating
- ○ Sweats
- ○ Cramping
- ○ Others:_____
- ○ _____

Bowel Movement

BM#1	BM#2	BM#3	BM#4
BM#5	BM#6	BM#7	BM#8

Energy Level   ○ Low   ○ Med   ○ High
Activity Level   ○ Low   ○ Med   ○ High
Mood   ○ Sad   ○ Good   ○ Happy

Sleep   ○ 😐   ○ 🙂

Notes: _____

Date:_____

S M T W T F S

Meals

Exercise:_____

Total Calories Burned:_____

Water Intake

	Time	Food & Drinks	Symptoms	Triggers	Notes
Breakfast					

Carb:_____, Fat:_____, Total Sugar:_____,
Fiber: _____, Protein:_____, Calories:_____

Snack					

Carb:_____, Fat:_____, Total Sugar:_____,
Fiber: _____, Protein:_____, Calories:_____

Lunch					

Carb:_____, Fat:_____, Total Sugar:_____,
Fiber: _____, Protein:_____, Calories:_____

Snack					

Carb:_____, Fat:_____, Total Sugar:_____,
Fiber: _____, Protein:_____, Calories:_____

Dinner					

Carb:_____, Fat:_____, Total Sugar:_____,
Fiber: _____, Protein:_____, Calories:_____

Pain

 How severe is the pain?

1   2   3   4   5

_____

_____

Did you take any medication?_____

Did it help?_____

Where does it hurt?

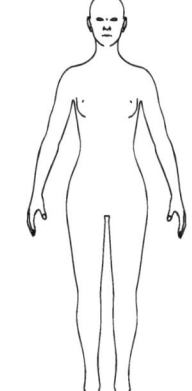

Time	Symptoms	Triggers

Other Symptoms Tracker

- O Pain
- O Constipation
- O Bleeding
- O Fatigue
- O Bloating
- O Sweats
- O Cramping
- O Others:_____
- O _____

Bowel Movement

BM#1	BM#2	BM#3	BM#4
BM#5	BM#6	BM#7	BM#8

Energy Level   O Low   O Med   O High

Activity Level   O Low   O Med   O High

Mood   O Sad   O Good   O Happy

Sleep   O   O

Notes:
_____

Date:_____

S M T W T F S

Meals

Exercise:_____

Total Calories Burned:_____

Water Intake

	Time	Food & Drinks	Symptoms	Triggers	Notes
Breakfast					

Carb:_____, Fat:_____, Total Sugar:_____,
Fiber: _____, Protein:_____, Calories:_____

Snack					

Carb:_____, Fat:_____, Total Sugar:_____,
Fiber: _____, Protein:_____, Calories:_____

Lunch					

Carb:_____, Fat:_____, Total Sugar:_____,
Fiber: _____, Protein:_____, Calories:_____

Snack					

Carb:_____, Fat:_____, Total Sugar:_____,
Fiber: _____, Protein:_____, Calories:_____

Dinner					

Carb:_____, Fat:_____, Total Sugar:_____,
Fiber: _____, Protein:_____, Calories:_____

Pain

Where does it hurt?

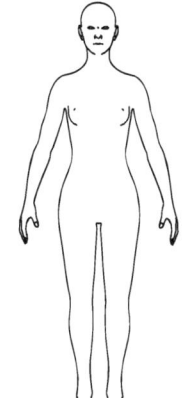

 How severe is the pain?

1　　2　　3　　4　　5

_____

_____

Did you take any medication? _____

Did it help? _____

Time	Symptoms	Triggers

Other Symptoms Tracker

- O Pain
- O Constipation
- O Bleeding
- O Fatigue
- O Bloating
- O Sweats
- O Cramping
- O Others:_____
- O _____

Bowel Movement

BM#1	BM#2	BM#3	BM#4
BM#5	BM#6	BM#7	BM#8

Energy Level　O Low　O Med　O High

Activity Level　O Low　O Med　O High

Mood　O Sad　O Good　O Happy

Sleep　O 　O

Notes: _____

We are so thrilled you've chosen to purchase our book. We hope you love it! If you do, would you consider posting an Online review on Amazon. This will help us to continue providing great products and helps potential buyers to make confident decisions.

Want free goodies?
Email us: Blackforestpublications@gmail.com

BLACK FOREST PUBLICATIONS

black_forest_publications

BLACK FOREST PUBLICATIONS

Amazon Author Page: Black Forest Publications

Copyright© 2021 Black Forest Publications

All rights reserved. No part of this publication may be reproduced, distributed, or transmitted in any form or by any mean including photocopying, recording, or other electronic or mechanical methods without the prior written permission of the author or publisher except in the case of brief quotations embodied in the critical reviews and certain other non - commercial uses permitted by the copyright law.
Please note that this medical logbook does not replace or replace or recommend any medical advice. Consult your medical institutions and physicians before taking any medication or action that involves your health.

Printed in Great Britain
by Amazon